The Ultimate
Getting Pregnant Fast Guide

Everything You Need to Know to Optimize Ovulation and Get Pregnant Faster

Kristina Duclos

Table of Contents

Introduction

I want to thank you and congratulate you for purchasing this book.

There are a million of couples out there who are trying to get pregnant for a long time. Hence, if you are one of this million, remember that you are not alone! This reference book is going to help you!

It is true that it takes time to conceive a child in the womb. Being fertile at the right moment is not an easy proposition. There are other concerns that you have to take into consideration. As such, everybody advises you that it would be very important to exercise patience. According to them, getting pregnant is not similar to turning on the switch of the light bulb. This is not untrue. However, patience, although a good and solid advice, may not be enough.

The reason for this is that there are many factors that determine whether you will get pregnant in this month or not. The major factors are your health, ovulation and the sexual methods that you use. In this book, you will know how to optimize your chances of getting pregnant by properly caring for your health and nutrition, by tracking your ovulation, and by engaging in efficient sexual methods.

This book contains the most comprehensive optimization techniques of getting pregnant in order to help you in your personal goals. The goal of this book is to provide the reader with techniques, and strategies that they can readily perform. As such, the author of this book has made it possible to create a getting pregnant fast reference book that provides a good working knowledge of the fundamental concepts that is highly practical, instead of passive and abstract. Unnecessary jargon, together with vague terms and concepts, are avoided in order to make it simple and easy to apply. Moreover, effort has been done to make the getting pregnant fast reference book as intuitive and easy to learn as possible.

All in all, the methods that are outlined in this book will give you increased chances in getting pregnant soon. In fact, this book will provide you with the most sophisticated and efficient knowledge in terms of proper ovulation, nutrition and sexual methods that is already used by most health care professionals!

Thanks again for purchasing this book, I hope you enjoy it! Please take some time to stop by and LIKE our Facebook page: https://www.facebook.com/joypublishing

With gratitude,

Kristina Duclos

Chapter 1

The Fundamental Principles of Ovulation and Getting Pregnant

In this chapter you will learn:

- Understanding Ovulation

    o Basics of Ovulation

    o Ovulation Facts

    o Ovulation: Does it occur before or after your period?

- Fertile Window

- The Fertile Phase of Your Cycle

- Signs of Ovulation

Understanding Ovulation

To put it simply, there is a 12 to 24 hour period when a fertile egg cell can be fertilized by a sperm cell. This is called the window of conception. Take note however, that the window of conception (12 to 24 hour period) is *not* the only time when conception (and getting pregnant) is possible. Do you want to know why? The reason is that unlike the fertile egg cell that is only available for a limited time, the sperm is available at any period of time. In fact, a sperm cell can live and survive inside the female uterus for up to five days! This is the reason why conception (and getting pregnant) is possible even after the window of conception. This concept will be further discussed in the latter part of this chapter and in chapter 2.

Understanding ovulation and the window of conception is the most important knowledge in getting pregnant fast. The reason for its importance lies in the fact that: By having a good working knowledge of the fundamental principles of ovulation and the window of conception, you and your partner will be able to know when is the best time to engage in sexual intercourse in order to get pregnant. In other words, you and your partner will be able to schedule the engagement in sexual intercourse in a time that is the most optimal for conception or getting pregnant.

Basics of Ovulation

Scientifically speaking, ovulation is the point in time when a female egg cell was released from the ovary. Afterwards, the female egg cell will travel down the fallopian tube where it will wait its turn to be fertilized by a sperm cell. Now, during the period of ovulation, if an egg cell that has been successfully been fertilized by a sperm cell, the lining of the uterine wall will thicken in order to give way to pregnancy.

Ovulation Facts

1. The cycle of ovulation usually alternates between the two ovaries

2. It is not impossible for a female to have ovulation even if she was not able to experience her period during a month

3. Light bleeding may happen during the cycle of ovulation

4. Only 1 egg cell is usually released from the ovary during each ovulation cycle

5. The egg cell will be available for fertilization for a period of 12 to 24 hours.

Ovulation: Does it occur before or after your Period?

One of the most frequently asked question is where ovulation occurs before or after the period. Technically speaking, ovulation should happen around the 14 day period immediately preceding your period. Does this mean that the best time to engage in sexual intercourse is on day 14 before your period?

Take note that this period assumes that your monthly cycle is 28 days. However, it is important to take into consideration that no woman is similar to any other! Therefore, it will be possible that your monthly cycle is 32 instead of 28 days.

In other words, there is even a slim chance that ovulation will happen on day 14 of your monthly cycle. As such, your chance of getting pregnant during that time is also slim.

Fertile Window

The best time to engage in sexual intercourse is solely dependent on the cycle of your ovulation. According to a recent research conducted by experts in physiology and female anatomy, for each cycle, the chance of getting pregnant is for exactly 6 days. This is the Critical 6 Day Fertile Window. The Critical 6 Day Fertile Window includes the time that the female egg cell is immediately available for fertilization (for 12 to 24 hours) and the 5 days immediately preceding ovulation.

Outside the Critical 6 Day Fertile Window, the chances of getting pregnant is very slim. In other words, knowing your Critical 6 Day Fertile Window is very important. According to the said study, the best chance of getting pregnant is at the following times in relation to the day of ovulation:

1. The day 2 days immediately preceding the day of ovulation;

2. The day immediately preceding the day of ovulation;

3. The day of ovulation itself.

The Fertile Phase of Your Cycle

The Fertile Phase of your cycle should not be confused with the Critical 6 Day Fertile Window. The Fertile Phase refers to the days in your ovulation cycle in which you may be within the Critical 6 Day Fertile Window. In other words, the Critical 6 Day Fertile Window is inside the fertile phase. For most women, the fertile phase happens between Day 6 and Day 21 of your cycle (a total of 16 days). However, it would be important to take into consideration that if you have a history of cycles that are highly irregular, your fertile phase may be much longer than that mentioned. If that is the case, you can use the signs of ovulation discussed below in order to help you determine the time of your ovulation.

Signs of Ovulation

The cycle of ovulation differs from one woman to another. As such, the cycle of ovulation of your mother (during her younger years), your sister or your friend will not be similar to yours. However, the biological changes that happen to women during the cycle of ovulation is fairly similar for each woman. Therefore, the signs of ovulation are consistent. These signs of ovulation are more commonly referred to as the symptoms of ovulation.

Basically, there are two types of symptoms of ovulation:

1. Primary symptoms of ovulation;

2. Secondary symptoms of ovulation.

On the one hand, primary symptoms of ovulation refer to that type of symptoms that are experienced by all women and can readily be spotted. The primary symptoms of ovulation are the following:

- Basal body temperature spike

- Cervical mucus becomes more slippery

- Cervical position becomes more firm

On the other hand, secondary symptoms of ovulation refer to that type of symptoms that may not be experienced by all women. In addition, these symptoms are not easily recognizable. The secondary symptoms of ovulation are the following:

- Bloating

- Increased sexual urge or libido

- Sense of smell are heightened

- Sense of touch are heightened

- Sense of taste are heightened

- Light spotting

- Tenderness of the breasts

- Cramping

- Pain on one side

Remember that as a woman, you may or may not notice the secondary symptoms of ovulation. Not noticing the secondary symptoms is perfectly fine. However, if you do notice these types of symptoms, you can have an additional guide in order to track your ovulation. Tracking of the cycle of ovulation is discussed thoroughly in the succeeding chapter, A Guide on Optimizing Your Chances of Getting Pregnant by Tracking Your Ovulation.

Chapter 2

A Guide on Optimizing Your Chances of Getting Pregnant by Tracking Your Ovulation

In this chapter you will learn:

- Key Concepts in Getting Pregnant

- The Simple Calendar Method

- Natural Family Planning (Fertility Awareness)

- Ovulation Tests and Monitors

Key Concepts in Getting Pregnant

Once you know your period of ovulation, it will be relatively easier for you and your partner to create a schedule on when to engage in sexual intercourse. The problem however is that tracking your ovulation will not be easy, if not difficult. In this chapter, different ways on how to track your ovulation are outlined in order to help you reach your goal of getting pregnant fast.

However, keep in mind that it would be your and your partner's job to preserve the spontaneity and romance in your loving relationship. The reason is that many couples who have been struggling to get pregnant in the past have made sex more of a chore than an expression of mutual love and care. As such, it would be crucial to avoid thinking that you are engaging in sexual intercourse for the sole reason of getting pregnant.

As previously stated in the first chapter, the 12 to 24 hour window of conception is the period when your fertile egg cell will be ready to be fertilized by the sperm cell of your partner. Also, it has been stated that the sperm cell of your partner can live inside your uterus for a period of 5 days. This is the main reason why the Critical 6 Day Fertile Window is 6 days and not 12 to 24 hours. Now, the question is this: How can you take advantage of this fact?

Remember that there is a greater chance of conception and getting pregnant when:

- The sperm cell is waiting inside the female uterus for the egg cell (during the Critical 6 Day Fertile Window); compared when

- It is the egg cell that is waiting to be fertilized by the sperm cell (during the exact point of ovulation).

Do you know the reason? It is because the first option provides you and your partner with a lot more flexibility and leeway (6 days) as compared to trying to precisely time your engagement in sexual intercourse at the exact point of ovulation (12 to 24 hours).

You may now be asking on what are the ways on which you can efficiently track your ovulation. To put it simply, there are 2 basic ways on which you can track your ovulation:

1. Using the calendar method (will be discussed shortly)

2. Using the primary and secondary symptoms of ovulation (as discussed in the first chapter).

Apart from the calendar method and the symptoms of ovulation, there are alternative ways and methods in which you can track your ovulation. These alternative ways are:

- Natural Family Planning (Fertility Awareness; and

- Ovulation Tests and Monitors.

Both of these methods will be discussed below.

The Simple Calendar Method

Actually, there are a lot of calendar based methods that are specifically designed to determine the exact time of ovulation. These methods include the following:

❖ Standard Days Method

❖ Modified Standard Days Method

❖ Rhythm Method

❖ The Simple Calendar Method

The Standard Days Method, Modified Standard Days Method, and the Rhythm Method are not discussed in this work because they are complicated in the sense that they will require you to make calculations solely based on the tracking period that you did for several months at a time. Also, most of them are based on flawed assumptions. In other words, should you use them, there is a chance that you might be missing out on key opportunities for getting pregnant each month. As such, it is believed that the simple calendar method is the best calendar method that you can use in order to determine the exact point or time of your ovulation.

In Simple Calendar Method, you will simply count 10 days immediately succeeding the first day you bleed. The first day you bleed refers to the first day of your monthly menstruation cycle. Now, what you will do is to engage in sexual intercourse with your partner every other day until the 21st day of your menstruation cycle.

In this way, you will be able to take advantage of the Critical 6 Day Fertile Window. In addition, there will also be some 'leeway days'. The reason for the existence of the 'leeway days' is that the exact point or time of your ovulation may vary from one month to another. Hence, taking into consideration the aforementioned variances, it would be prudent to include some 'leeway days' into the Critical 6 Day Fertile Window.

Natural Family Planning (Fertility Awareness)

Natural Family Planning refers to the practice of determining the exact day of your ovulation through the following means:

- Monitoring your temperature using a basal thermometer; and

- Checking your cervical mucus

The purpose of monitoring your temperature using a basal thermometer is that such thermometer is very sensitive and will reflect a sudden increase in your temperature that happens during the day of your ovulation.

The purpose of checking your cervical mucus is that during the period of your ovulation, the cervical mucus becomes more slippery, wet, and elastic. In addition, you will notice that your cervical mucus has the capability of being stretched between your fingers if you pull them apart and press them together. Some women described the texture of the cervical mucus during the period of ovulation as similar to egg whites.

Ovulation Tests and Monitors

Ovulation Tests and Monitors refers to a series test strips which is used in order to determine the surge of Luteinizing Hormone (LH) in your urine immediately preceding the period of ovulation.

The best thing about using these Ovulation Tests and Monitors is that the surge of Luteinizing Hormone (LH) in your urine happens during the 3 days immediately preceding the period of ovulation. As already stated, this 3 day window is one of the best times for conception. The reason for this is that such 3 day period is *well within* the Critical 6 Day Fertile Window. In other words, by using the ovulation test and monitor strips, it will be relatively easier for you and your partner to schedule the time for engagement in sexual intercourse that has the best chance of conceiving a child!

Chapter 3

A Guide on Optimizing Your Chances of Getting Pregnant Through Sexual Methods

In this chapter you will learn:

- The Best Sexual Position to Increase the Chances of Getting Pregnant

- Frequency of Sexual Intercourse

- Timing of Sexual Intercourse

- Things That You Should Never Do

The Best Sexual Position to Increase the Chances of Getting Pregnant

You might be wondering, "Is there a correct and incorrect way in performing sexual intercourse?" The answer is a simple no. The fact of the matter is you can get pregnant with *any* sexual position. Remember that as long as the sperm cell meets the egg cell, conception is possible. In other words, as long as there is contact of the semen of your partner in your vagina, there is a chance of getting pregnant. As such, it may be more important for you to use your efforts in the making sure that the sperm cells of your partner are of utmost health.

However, if there is one sexual position that you can use in order to maximize the chances of getting pregnant – such sexual position is the 'missionary style' where your partner will be on top and while you are lying on the bed. The reason is that the semen will be in the best position to reach the innermost part of your vagina (your uterus) immediately after ejaculation. In addition, it would be even better if you can use the modified missionary style sexual position where your partner is on top while you are lying on the bed with your legs elevated over his shoulders. In this way, you will be greatly aided by gravity and it also allows for deepest penetration.

Thus, the 'missionary style,' as far as the other sexual positions are concerned, is the best sexual position to increase your chances of getting pregnant.

Frequency of Sexual Intercourse

The frequency of sexual intercourse is an important component of getting pregnant fast. The reason for this is that the frequency of sexual intercourse will directly affect the quantity and quality of your partner's sperm cells. To put it simply:

1. On the one hand, if the frequency of sexual intercourse is too low (i.e., over the span of one week, he was not able to ejaculate), the seminal fluid will be filled with a good number of damaged and dead sperm cells.

2. On the other hand, if the frequency of sexual intercourse is too high (i.e., over the span of one week, he was able to ejaculate every day), the seminal fluid will be filled with a good number of immature and young sperm cells.

In both cases, the seminal fluid will not be as effective in conceiving a child. The recommended frequency of sexual intercourse is every other day during your fertile phase. In this way, you and your partner will be able to maximize the full quality and quantity of the sperm cells that is potent for fertilization. If you and your partner cannot manage to have sexual intercourse every other day, then every three days will also be optimal.

Timing of Sexual Intercourse

The time when men are most fertile is during the morning after a good sleep the night before. Hence, it is during the morning when men have the most quantity of sperm cells available. Therefore, it would make sense to schedule your sexual intercourse during the morning immediately after waking up.

Things That You Should Never Do

There are 5 things that you should never do if you want to optimize the chances of conception and getting pregnant. These are the following:

1. Avoid taking medications such as antihistamines. Although antihistamines might solve your problem with colds, it was found that they can also dry up your cervical mucus. Dry cervical mucus will prevent the sperm cells from reaching your uterus.

2. Do not engage in sexual intercourse while in a hot tub. Remember that high temperature quickly kills sperm cells.

3. Most commercially available lubricants today contain spermicides. As such, you have to avoid using them. However, should you really need lubricants, make sure that they do not contain spermicides by reading their contents.

4. Do not engage in sexual intercourse while bathing. Extreme temperatures, together with soap can kill the sperm cells.

5. Remind your partner that he should avoid using the laptop before engaging in sexual intercourse. The sperm cells are going to get killed from the heat of the laptop when placed near the groin area. However, should he really need to make use of the laptop, make sure that he puts the laptop on the table instead onto his lap.

Chapter 4

A Comprehensive Health and Nutrition Checklist during Conception

In this chapter you will learn:

- Nutrition and its importance

- Foods that you need to avoid

- Foods that you need to consume

Nutrition and its importance

When couples are trying to get pregnant, one of the questions that they frequently ask is: "Are there any foods that I can consume in order to help me get pregnant faster?" The answer is yes. Conversely, there are foods that you should avoid if you really want to get pregnant faster.

Good nutrition is synonymous with fertility. Therefore, eating well-balanced meals, eating the right kinds of foods, and avoiding the wrong kinds of foods will provide you with good health.

One of the best ways to increase the likelihood of getting pregnant is to invest in your health and well-being. Remember that a healthy body will enable you to do things that you want. One of those is trying to get pregnant. Conversely, if you are not presently healthy, your chances of getting pregnant may be low. In addition your good health at the time of conception will enhance the health and wellness of your future child in your womb.

Foods that you need to avoid

1. Caffeine

• According to research, caffeine can effectively lower your fertility by 27%.

• Apart from lowering your fertility, caffeine also hinders your body from absorbing essential nutrients such as calcium and iron.

2. Red Meat

• According to research, red meat can effectively cause endometriosis. As such, red meat is a risk in lowering your levels of fertility.

• In other words, it would be beneficial to limit your intake of red meat as much as possible.

3. Processed Foods

• Many commercial processed foods today actually contain a lot of preservatives, artificial hormones and even pesticides. As such, apart from causing obesity, processed foods are very harmful by significantly decreasing the levels of your hormonal health.

• Therefore you should avoid eating chips, frozen meals, cookies and other related food items such as hotdogs, bacon and sausage.

• Instead, you should consume foods that are organic. This includes fresh vegetables and fruits.

4. Soy Products

• According to recent studies, products that are based on soy have been consistently shown to significantly diminish the sperm counts in men. The culprit is the isoflavone compound called Genistein. Genistein are seen to slow and destroy the sperm cells inside the human body.

• As such, you should ask your partner to avoid (at least while you are trying to get pregnant) products that are based on soy such as edmame, soy milk and tofu.

5. Simple Carbohydrates and Refined Sugars

• One of the reasons why simple carbohydrates and refined sugars must be avoided is that these kinds of foods cause weight gain and obesity. Remember that couples who are overweight are definitely less fertile compared to their slimmer counterparts.

• In addition, simple carbohydrates and refined sugars also cause your body to use up more nutrients in order to process them.

• As such, you should avoid eating foods such as sweets, sugar, white flour, white pastas, and other refined grains.

6. Bad Fats

- It is important to take into consideration that there are two kinds of fats – the good fats and the bad fats. Good fats are the kinds of fats that you should not avoid such as mono unsaturated fats found in olive oil.

- On the other hand, the fats that you should avoid are the bad fats. Bad fats are consistently found to decrease the levels of your fertility. Bad fats are:

  - partially hydrogenated fats (trans fats) found in processed foods; and

  - saturated fats found in red meat

Foods That You Need to Consume

1. Water

- Water is very important to enable your organs to function more effectively. This is because water have a specific mechanism to help deliver the nutrients that you intake from food toward the rest of your body.

- In addition, remember that hormones are very important in pregnancy. It is consistently found by science that water causes hormonal balance throughout the body.

- Water also helps clear out the toxins out of your system.

2. Complex Carbohydrates

• Complex carbohydrates have nutrients that are favorable for pregnancy. In addition, complex carbohydrates also have fiber that is known to effectively remove the toxins out of your body.

• As such, remember to always consume carbohydrates such as brown rice, whole grain cereals, whole grain pasta, and vegetables.

3. Protein

• Protein is a nutrient that has a mechanism that contributes significantly in the production of hormones. As you now, hormones are very important in getting pregnant.

• The most healthy type of proteins are those found in foods such as oily fish, white meat, nuts, beans, seeds, and fresh eggs.

4. Whole Milk

• According to recent studies, drinking whole milk significantly increases the levels of fertility in women. According to the same research, women who drank at least 2 glasses of whole milk during the period of ovulation are 70% more likely to get pregnant.

• The reason, according to the researchers, is that whole milk contains natural hormones that boost the fertility of women.

• As such, it would be beneficial if you consume whole milk while you are trying to get pregnant.

Conclusion

Thank you again for purchasing this book!

Most likely, this getting pregnant fast reference book has provided you with ideas on how to increase your odds of getting pregnant soon!

I hope this book was able to help you to know the optimized techniques and strategies with respect to ovulation, nutrition and sexual methods with the goal of helping you get pregnant fast!

The next step you have to take in getting pregnant fast is to apply this knowledge every day (with respect to nutrition and the sexual methods) and every menstrual cycle (with respect to ovulation). Be sure to re-read it on a regular basis to remind yourself and make the most of it in your life! Soon enough, you will have that 'positive' result on your pregnancy test!

Finally, please remember to check out our Facebook page in order to find other resources and upcoming promotions:

https://www.facebook.com/joypublishing

With sincere thanks,

Kristina Duclos

Preview Of "How to Predict Your Baby Gender: Guide to Fertility and Achieving the Baby Gender of Your Dreams"

Introduction

Dear Reader,

Thank you for purchasing *"How to Predict Your Baby Gender."* I feel so privileged to share my years of knowledge and experience with you in this informational and practical book.

I am the mother of a toddler and have personal experience with baby gender prediction techniques. I was successful in predicting the gender of my baby girl the moment I found out I was pregnant: over 15 weeks before any ultrasound test! I only officially confirmed her gender when she was born. During those eight months, I was confident that I was having a girl; I even went as far as purchasing a few butterfly and flower decorations for her nursery.

My hope is that through this book you will apply these prediction techniques to your own experience and find the same success that I did. Share my journey of birth control and pregnancy with me. Afterwards, learn the techniques for predicting your baby's gender. Finally, apply the techniques in your own life to create your own story. Even though Mother Nature will always make her plans, we are still able to swing the decision in a more favorable direction.

Enjoy,

Kristina Duclos

Chapter 1 - How It All Started: My Personal Journey

I easily get excited and passionate when talking about baby gender prediction techniques. I love sharing the information with anyone who will listen. Furthermore, I love impressing people with my own success of predicting my daughter's gender. This knowledge and experience that I gained about predicting baby gender originally came from a fantastic fertility awareness book that changed my life: Taking Charge of Your Fertility by Toni Weschler.

I was first introduced to the concepts of baby gender prediction and fertility awareness when I was switching from the birth control pill to some kind of natural method. I wasn't thrilled with the birth control pill. I believe that it altered my personality and made me feel "crazy." I was originally planning to switch to a different pill until I started reading Toni Weschler's book. It forever changed my attitude towards birth control and convinced me of the benefits of a more natural approach.

As I learned more about the intricacies of the female body, I developed a deep respect and awe for how the female body was built. At this point in time, I knew that I no longer wanted to use the birth control pill, even if I found one that was a better fit. On the contrary, I wanted to experience the ups and downs of my fertility cycle the way nature intended it to be. No more pills or synthetic hormones for me.

Once I taught myself how to read my body's fertility signs, I discovered the fascinating facts about baby gender prediction. I soon got pregnant and had the opportunity to interpret these facts in my own pregnancy. Although I never confirmed my baby's gender until after she was born, I knew her gender from day one based on the gender prediction techniques. It was as clear as day that I was having a girl.

Chapter 2 - Why Fertility Awareness and Not Some Other Natural Method?

Before I was ready to get pregnant, I needed to find a birth control method that I was satisfied with. During my journey to find something natural, I considered a few options: IUDs, condoms and withdrawal. As soon as I read Toni Wechler's book, I knew that natural birth control was the way for me. I had enough respect for my cycle that I no longer wanted to manipulate it.

Click here to check out the rest of this book on Amazon.

Or go to: http://amzn.to/1pdOPiG

Check Out My Other Books

Below you'll find some of my other books that are popular on Amazon and Kindle as well. You can visit my author page on Amazon to see other work done by me. Alternatively, you can simply search for these titles on the Amazon website to find them.

Fertility: Getting Pregnant Fast - Guide to Everything You Need to Know to Optimize Ovulation & Get Pregnant Faster

Family Planning: Fertility, Get Pregnant & How to Predict Your Baby Gender

Diaper Free: Baby Guide - Elimination Communication Strategies for Quicker & Healthier Potty Training Before 18 Months

One Last Thing...

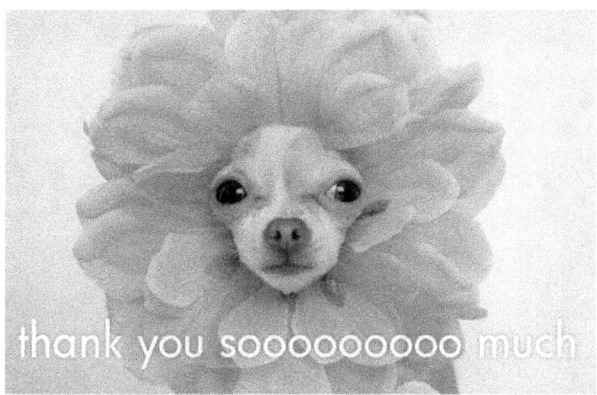

thank you sooooooooo much

If you believe that this book is worth sharing, would you please take the time to let others know how it affected your life? If it turns out to make a difference in the lives of others, they will be forever grateful to you, as will I.